Get Inside Her: 30 Dirty Tips to Help You Seduce and Get Her in Bed on the First Date

Disclaimer and Terms of Use: Effort has been made to ensure that the information in this book is accurate and complete, however, the author and the publisher do not warrant the accuracy of the information, text and graphics contained within the book due to the rapidly changing nature of science, research, known and unknown facts and internet. The Author and the publisher do not hold any responsibility for errors, omissions or contrary interpretation of the subject matter herein. This book is presented solely for motivational and informational purposes only.

Table of Contents

Introduction

Seducing a young woman could be simple, yet troublesome, contingent upon how you take a gander at it. Assuming that you think that it simple, that is since you has had a few experiences. Anyhow assuming that you think that it troublesome, chances are, you're even now feeling your path around, and attempting distinctive techniques to see what lives up to expectations.

Forgot to tell you one more thing; do not forget, or divert from your motive at any cost which few men do, they create a mystery while seducing their partner. Always use pun while speaking with her as conversation is the best way to seduce a girl. The foremost thing you should understand is the need of your partner, though it is difficult for a person to read women's mind.

When I begin I need to verify you comprehend the distinction between tempting a young woman and badgering her or far more detestable striking her. In the event that the young woman you are attempting to tempt is unmistakably not intrigued or appears uncomfortable top whatever you do at that instant.

- Seducing a woman is like hitting the dance floor with a woman. Frequently you hold her nearby and at times, you give her a chance to sparkle on her own and watch. Assuming that you are excessively clingy, she will feel suffocated.

Assuming that you release her and never return, she will be offended.

- In the event that she faculties that you are alluring her, she will flee. The pace of your enchantment ought to be abated and the volume ought to be peaceful.

- In the event that you finished something remarkably wrong, apologize rapidly and truly. Recognize her side of the story with a beguiling, receptive straightforwardness. Ladies like compassion and encouraging from men they are intrigued by.

- Compassion is crucial to enchantment. Each lady is distinctive, so tailor your date, your words and your movements to that particular lady. You must comprehend what she is thinking before you can offer her the joy she wants.

- Uncover yourself gradually and just when specifically asked. Don't demonstrate a greater amount of yourself than she requests. The point when the secret is gone, the enchantment loses its value.

- Assuming that you need to lure a young woman, the first thing you have to do is improve. Do not go ahead excessively solid or she would feel debilitated or discover you excessively simple to get, and may get exhausted of you.

- The ideal approach to get mischievous and private with a woman is by messaging her late during the evening, or by ringing her when she is sleeping. Begin by messaging late in the nighttime in the first place, and inside a day or two, she may be agreeable enough to content you or talk with you late into the night regardless of the possibility that she is uncomfortable with the thought from the beginning.

- In view of my experience with young women, I have created a standard pattern for my dates. The triumph rate is greatly high, to such an extent that I might even say its idiot proof. Right away, here it is:

- The principal thing you have to do his methodology. As if they say with the lottery, you cannot win in the event that you do not play. Approaching is just troublesome assuming that you have not destroyed it a while. When you get over your starting dread, you will observe that it is simple. The women, which used to threaten you, now appear as though jokes.

This is not the exercise on approaching. I am accepting that you can get a date at any rate of time. It does not make a difference how, if it were from the Internet through a companion or by icy methodologies. When you have the date, this is the point at which the fun starts.

- Ask your date to reach you at an unbiased area close to your house. When you go out to reach her, let her know you are simply getting a few things together. Walk her once again to your house. Surely, you will have cleaned beforehand. The reason for carrying her to your house is to get her acclimated to being there.

Later on, when you welcome her again for some espresso, she will have been in your condominium and will be more open to backpedaling.

- The point when the two of you backtrack, make certain to have your rucksack pressed with if the materials recorded previously. You would prefer not to stay excessively long, sufficiently yearn for you to get the pack and take off.

- When you have left, move ahead to the area of the date. I exceedingly encourage you to pick an isolates area, for example, the shore, a recreation center, or something to that effect.

- Indeed a cemetery might be fine. At whatever point you do, to not head off to a bar, pub, or club. Not just will this revive memories in the young women brain of irregular fellows hitting on her, yet it will likewise place you in the class of gentlemen who don't make a decent attempt when going on dates.

- By picking a separated area, you will likewise dispose of any preoccupations regularly connected with normal nightlife foundations i.e. No noisy music, no different young women to gaze at, and no different fellows hitting on your woman. Just you and your date in a private area, where you can get to know each other.

- By and by, I live by the sunny shore, with the goal that where my dates happen. When you arrive, evacuate the sheet or cover and ask your date to bail you spread it out. Captivating her in the movement of the date will mentally make her imagine that she has put a greater amount of herself in it.

- Make an astounding impression come what may. Initial introductions matter. In opposition to prevalent thinking, however, you do not just get one initial introduction in every relationship. Think about every time you see her, discussion to her, or generally cooperate with her in the wake of being truant as another early introduction, and make it a great one.

When you lift her up for a date, look cleaned, and pay her an astonishing compliment. "You look staggering" normally works well.

- When you get the telephone, grin and say "Hey, perfect." She cannot see you grin, yet she will have the capacity to hear it in your voice, trust me.

- When you message or IM her, do not start only with "hey" or "howdy." There's no substance there. Say something like, "I can't quit contemplating you" or "How my most is loved young lady on the planet today?"

- Clean yourself up. You most likely know this, yet most women think a ton about hygiene. Do not stress over using throughout the day preparing — an additional 5 or 10 minutes added to your common routine can have a universe of effect. Begin with these:

- Make your mouth as engaging as could reasonably be expected. Always brush, floss, and use mouthwash in any event twice a day. Assuming that you have to spruce up after a feast, utilize gum or mints.

- Maintain a strategic distance from sharp nourishments like garlic and onions for a day or two preceding you see your darling. Not just do they make your mouth horrible, the aroma really leaves your sweat organs for a couple of days after you consume. Furthermore, nobody needs onion sweat.

- Shower as frequently as you have to. You ought to be hitting one shower a day at any rate, yet make it more assuming that you have a tendency to get filthy. Only got back from work and now you possess a scent reminiscent of food/cars/office supplies. Shower. You get the thought.

Staying as clean as would be prudent keeps you primed for a minute ago experiences. Imagine a scenario where she needs to drop abruptly by your house since she was in the region. Suppose it is possible that she calls and needs to head off to a motion picture that begins in 10 minutes. Assuming that you are as of now clean, you are great to head off at whatever point you have to.

- Deal with your facial hair. You might be clean-shaven, or you can have genuine whiskers. Being anywhere amidst and having scruff is not exactly perfect. Shave scruff, trim facial hair. It is done.

Trim and clean your nails. Make a propensity of cutting your fingernails and toenails each few days, when you escape the shower. Both ought to be trimmed short enough that there's just a flimsy line of white between the closure of the nail and the snappy.

- Freshen up. Slap on some antiperspirant the second you escape the shower, and reapply as frequently as you have to throughout the day. Put on a most extreme of two squirts of cologne for additional exertion. **(Note that exaggerating cologne might be more terrible than not wearing cologne — go simple.)**

- Converse with her, Inquiry: What is the greatest human sexual organ? Reply: The mind. When you do all else, you need to help her believe that you are somebody she needs to have alluring her. A great deal of that recognition will be colored by what you discuss, so here's a snappy first stage:

Do discuss:

1. How astonishing you think she is
2. Her hobbies
3. What she needs out of what's to come
4. What you need out of what's to come
5. Imparted encounters or different things you have in like manner

Do not discuss:

1. The old stand-bys: cash, legislative issues, and religion
2. Other ladies
3. Crap jokes
4. Why your life sucks and how it's never set to improve
5. Things that you know she discovers hostile

- Do take the time to pay her a ravishing compliment occasionally. Consider something you truly like or respect about this young woman and expression it in the most honest to goodness and complimenting way you can. Assuming that you can do this right a couple times, she will liquefy.

- Do discuss sex in a stately manner, in the event that it commonly comes up in the discussion. Be unobtrusive about recognizing your sexual side — you would prefer not to threaten her, however you likewise do not need her to overlook that it is there. Case in point, you could say "Slumber is my second most loved thing to do in bunk" or "I may require a frosty shower in the event that you continue talking like that."

Set the mind-set. Assuming that you can control nature's turf whatsoever, taking these little steps will help the climate appear to be more attractive and private.

- Keep the lighting faint. In the event that you are at home, utilize delicate lights, or light a few candles.

- Deal with the temperature. In the event that it is a bit cold, you will have the chance to give her your coat or have her cuddle up to you.

- Make it a sheltered space. "Sheltered" as in, a range where she feels great being near you. Sitting in your filthy loft while your flat mate noisily examines football does not check.

- Touch her in little, enchanting ways. Yes, you will most likely be the one to break the touch restraint. However, you can do it. It is simpler than it appears. Here are a couple of prescriptions for distinctive circumstances:

- In the event that you are standing or strolling, rest your hand on the little of her back (where her spine bends internal, simply above her butt). Keep your weight light and delicate. This is an improved elective to carelessly tossing your arm around her shoulders.

Assuming that you are sitting alongside her, softly rest your hand on her knee for a couple of seconds. This is best assuming that you do it while you are conversing with her, so both of you are not clumsily viewing you touch her and move away. Give it a chance to wait for a minute while you keep on speaking, and then gradually pull it back.

- Assuming that she is standing near you put your arm around her waist. Rest your hand (once more, softly) simply above her hip, in the bend of her waist.

- Do not only run with the adage arm-around-the-shoulders. Rather, wrap your arm down her back, so your hand is resting where her shoulder reaches her neck. In the event that that appears as though its going great, you can delicately run your thumb over the once again of her neck.

Offer her a foot rub or shoulder rub. Most individuals, without taking into consideration most women, will not turn down a free back rub. In the event that you are in a cool setting where this is conceivable, such as sitting on the love seat viewing a film, make every effort to impress.

- In the event that you are providing for her a foot rub, concentrate on one foot at once. Support it in both hands, and keep your developments moderate while applying medium weight. Assuming that she shuts her eyes or sighs, you are completing it right.

- In the event that you are providing for her a shoulder rub, oppose the allurement to promptly put your fingers under her shirt, instead, utilize your thumbs on her exposed neck while your different fingers rest on her secured shoulders, practically touching her collarbones. Once more, keep your movements abate and point for medium weight.

Raise the stakes. In the event that the back rub is going great and you can let she know responsive, attempt extending your region. For example, in the event that you are providing for her a foot rub, attempt gradually climbing to her calves. Assuming that you are providing for her a shoulder rub, attempt moving you is undoubtedly her spine, keeping your thumbs concentrated on the muscles around it.

- Stop before she is primed for you. The focus here is to get her appreciating and needing your touch. In the event that you stop amidst a marvelous back rub, she will intuitively need to discover approaches to get the stimulation going once more. Time it with the goal that you know she is having a ball; however, she is no place close exhausted or satisfied.

Give her a chance to come to you. When you have broken the touch boundary and demonstrated to her you that are intrigued, it is on her to do a smidge of the work. Check whether she sits near you, pokes you, or overall rationalizes to touch you. In the event that she does, you are more right than wrong. If not, attempt returning to the past steps on more than one occasion and check whether that warms her up.

- Remember the "90-10 standard. You are ready to begin the collaboration and do 90% of the work, however she needs to reach you on the last 10%. Case in point, assuming that you go in for a kiss, you start it and move in a large portion of the way — however make it so she need to incline in the last little touch and really begin the kiss.

- Provide for her a sense-blowing kiss. In the event that every bit of her indicators so far has been sure, go in for the kiss. Amp up your common strategy by:

Keeping it light and moderate from the beginning will delicately brush your lips over hers on the first pass, and put your tongue away for the initial couple of kisses.

- Completing the right things with your hands- You could rest them gently in the bends of her waist, put them on her shoulders, or tangle them up in her hair and put them on the once more of her head. Each of the three is great.

Knowing when to move to French kissing- Begin by softly running your tongue over her base lip. In the event that she opens her mouth more, go in. If not, spare it for an alternate time.

- Concentrate on her erogenous zones. Erogenous zones are essentially territories on the physique where there are tons of nerve endings, making them touchier. Centering your consideration on them can bail you get more mileage out of a make-out. **Begin with light touches, and proceed onward to light kisses in the event that you think it's time:**

1. Throat, neck, jaw and collarbones
2. Ears
3. Within her arms
4. Wrists
5. Palms
6. Mid-region
7. Thighs (particularly inward thighs)
8. Feet and toes
9. Lower back

Clear regions: bum, breasts, and privates

I need to emphasize that these moves may as well just be made once you feel that this young woman is agreeable enough for you to take that jump. Assuming that she has consented to the date in any case, you have not botched it some way or another by appearing destitute, and there is no motivation behind why she should not.

- Besides, until you do this a few times, it may be challenging you to judge when the right minute to make a move is. Thusly, I suggest that you only try hard when you feel that the young woman is drawing in to you. Strike when the iron is hot, for example, in the wake of making her chuckle.

Expecting everything has worked out as expected and she is straddling you, do not hesitate to get more sexual with her. With the two of you in this position, sex is as of now on both of your psyches. Your employment as a man is to raise this sexual methodology to the focus where the young woman is prepared.

- Clearly, things like kissing, grabbing, in running your without a doubt the length of her constitution are incredible approaches to get her in the temperament. One extra trap which

I discovered works well is to lift up your shirt, and her shirt, with the goal that both of your stomachs are touching. This method will trigger memories of sexual encounters, pushing the young woman further into a sexual state.

You do not dependably need to strive for the grand slam. As it were not every date requirements to end in sex. There is nothing the matter with taking somewhat more of an opportunity to tempt the young woman.

- That being said, you have to lead the association to an enchantment area. The point when the young lady is sufficiently stimulated, propose that the two of you may as well about-face to your spot, **keeping in mind the end goal to:**

1. Watch a film
2. Hear some out music
3. Have some coffee/tea
4. Walk the pooch
5. Encourage the feline
6. Put your clothing in the dryer

- The thought is to recommend an honest movement, which only happens to be in the same room as your bunk. Assuming that you have done your occupation rightly and have sufficiently broken down her obstructions, then she will concur.

It is critical to make a note here that the best time to prescribe the skip to the temptation area is the point at which you perceive the young woman getting to be sexually stimulated. Assuming that you end up stuck in a marathon make out session, you know you held up excessively long.

- When you have stuffed up your stuff and are headed back, play it cool. In the event that you feel great enough, you can put your arm around her shoulder. A few young women like these others think that it uncomfortable. Do it at any rate. It demonstrates a certain level of certainty.

An alternate tip I might want to provide for you is to take a piss before you clear out. I will illustrate this in a minute.

- When you have returned to your loft, you should simply make a move. The young woman will likely need to go pee, yet attempt to make your turn before she goes. Keep the sexual vitality high.

This is the reason you might as well take a piss before you return home. Yes, it could be somewhat horrible piss before your date, assuming that you hold up until after she goes, then when you return to your room, you will have lost your force.

- Meanwhile, you can put some delicate music on. Have a condom close-by and tear the edge of the wrapper somewhat. There is nothing more regrettable than bobbling with a condom wrapper right before sex.

Summary

When she returns, you have to make a move once more. Begin by kissing her and putting your involved her constitution. After second, take off your shirt. The demonstration of uncovering is exceptionally sexual, so take off the same amount of your attire as you can. Help her take off her attire, as well.

www.ingramcontent.com/pod-product-compliance
Lightning Source LLC
Chambersburg PA
CBHW061951280526
45787CB00004B/1820